Asthma Help

Guide to Treatment Options, Tips and Lifestyle Adjustments for Managing Asthma and the Symptoms of Asthma So That You Can Live the Life You Want

By Jim Russlan

© **Copyright 2020 - All rights reserved.**

The content contained within this book may not be reproduced, duplicated or transmitted without direct written permission from the author or the publisher.

Under no circumstances will any blame or legal responsibility be held against the publisher or author for any damages, reparation, or monetary loss due to the information contained within this book. Either directly or indirectly.

Legal Notice:

This book is copyright protected. This book is only for personal use. You cannot amend, distribute, sell, use, quote or paraphrase any part, or the content within this book, without the consent of the author or publisher.

Disclaimer Notice:

Please note the information contained within this document is for educational and entertainment purposes only. All effort has been executed to present accurate, up to date and reliable, complete information. No warranties of any kind are declared or implied. Readers acknowledge that the author is not engaging in the rendering of legal, financial, medical or professional advice. The content within this book has been derived from various sources. Please consult a licensed professional before attempting any techniques outlined in this book.

By reading this document, the reader agrees that under no circumstances is the author responsible for any losses, direct or indirect, which are incurred as a result of the use of information contained within this document, including, but not limited to, —errors, omissions, or inaccuracies.

Contents

Introduction 1

Chapter 1: What is Asthma 2

Chapter 2: Asthma is More Than It Appears............................8

    Inflammatory Triggers. 9

    Asthma Triggers 14

    The List is Long 21

    Can Asthma Be Cured?...24

Chapter 2: Drugs 27

Chapter 3: Drugs for Long-Term Asthma Control 29

    What They Are and How They Function.........................29

    Side Effects 32

    Incorporating Natural Methods.......................................35

Chapter 4: Quick Fix Asthma Drugs..38

Chapter 5: Well-Managed Asthma 40

    Peak Flow Meter...40

    Spirometry 42

    Other Elements for Controlling Asthma 45

Chapter 6: Changing Your Lifestyle...47

Chapter 7: Natural Treatments 52

    Multivitamins 53

    Honey 54

    Garlic 55

    Apple Cider Vinegar...57

    Get Rid of Dairy..57

Remove Wheat (Gluten) Based Items 58

Drink Black Coffee 59

Take Cold Showers..59

Herbs 60

A Natural Asthma Eating Plan 64

Chapter 8: Less Known Natural Options..67

Halotherapy or Speleotherapy 67

Marine Phytoplankton 68

Embracing a Homeopathic Approach to Dealing With Asthma 70

Conclusion 73

Thank you for buying this book and I hope that you will find it useful. If you will want to share your thoughts on this book, you can do so by leaving a review on the Amazon page, it helps me out a lot.

Introduction

Have you or has anybody you know been diagnosed with asthma? If yes, you might be a bit baffled by the questions to which nobody appears to be able to provide an answer to.

As you are going to find as you go through this book, among the reasons why asthma victims frequently find themselves left in the dark regarding their issue is that even though the standard definition of asthma is extremely straightforward, nearly all else about the condition isn't.

Subsequently, in this book, I'm going to respond to as many asthma-related questions as I can. Then, I am going to introduce a range of natural treatments that are actually proven to be helpful in dealing with asthma.

Chapter 1: What is Asthma

The very first question to deal with is, "What is asthma?" Thankfully, this is the simplest of all the asthma questions, due to the fact that the medical profession in its entirety remains in broad agreement regarding how to categorize and describe asthma. At its core, physicians agree that asthma is a breathing condition that leads to 'chronic swelling of the air passages.'

Individuals frequently show signs well before asthma establishes itself since asthma could begin with something as simple as a cough or cold. Other signs that might point to asthma consist of moderate shortness of breath, sneezing, and even something outside your respiratory tract or lungs like a headache.

The bottom line is that it is very common for the preliminary indications of asthma to be neglected due to the fact that they seem like nothing more than the signs of a typical, everyday condition like a cold or a cough. This absence of awareness is among the primary reasons why many individuals do not look for asthma treatment.

Asthma Society of Canada claims that as many as 6 out of every 10 Canadians who have asthma do not manage their condition. This figure is anticipated to be comparable in other industrialized Western countries.

Since asthma is a chronic condition, it is one which needs to be handled during your life. It induces swelling, and for that reason, tightens the air passages that bring air in your lungs. Subsequently, this limits the air passage from the outside world through an asthma victim's lungs, rendering it challenging for them to breathe.

Asthma victims' air passages are sensitive to lots of conditions, like warm, moist, or cold air, irritants, tension, or physical exertion. The muscles which surround the air passages respond to these conditions by tightening and contracting the air passages of an individual with asthma.

The issue is normally intensified by the reality that the muscles additionally induce excess mucous to be generated during the contraction, additionally obstructing the air passages.

Nevertheless, a lot of the most typical indications of an asthma attack could frequently be acknowledged well before the condition itself is established. A few of the indications of asthma are apparent, whereas others may not be as quickly acknowledged, and potentially, they may be the outcome of another medical condition. The less apparent the signs are, the less advanced the asthma is, and it is less probable that the signs are going to develop into asthma.

Less intense indications that may fall into the 'early warning' group might consist of any of the following:

- Regular changes of mood

- Regular sneezing bouts

- Watery or Glassy eyes

- Dry mouth

- Uneasiness

- Sleeping troubles

- Unexplained increased fatigue

- Dark circles beneath the eyes

- Persistent or continuous headaches

- Exercise intolerance

- Pale skin tone

Clearly, all of these 'early warning' indications might recommend that asthma may end up being an issue, however, they might additionally be the outcome of another severe medical condition.

As a result, you would not always presume that any of the signs in the prior list are a clear precursor or sign of asthma. Nevertheless, if these signs are disregarded, the condition is very likely to intensify for anybody who is at risk of establishing asthma.

When the condition intensifies, the signs end up being significantly apparent. These signs might consist of:

- Shortness of breath, specifically after basic exercise like strolling or climbing up the stairs

- Coughing, wheezing and overall chest tightness

- Inability to think plainly

- Inability to talk

- Apparent nasal flaring as they strain to breathe in

- Sagging posture or hunched shoulders suggesting which the victim is straining for breath

- A grey or grey-blue tint slowly appearing on the skin, typically beginning around the mouth and nose part

- A contraction in part beneath the ribs and in the neck while straining to breathe

Any of these indications would be a sign of what we would generally acknowledge as an 'asthma attack.'

Everything about asthma up to this point appears fairly simple since you are going to most likely acknowledge asthma 'signs' - particularly if you know somebody who struggles with the condition. Asthma is a remarkably typical condition and one which the majority of us are familiar with to certain extent.

Chapter 2: Asthma is More Than It Appears

There are numerous elements which make asthma an incredibly intricate issue as well as an easy one, elements which suggest that there are likely no two individuals who have precisely the identical type of asthma.

While we do know that asthma is going to normally be seen in young people initially, medical science is still not able to separate precisely what induces asthma. What researchers have actually been able to figure out is that asthma could establish due to hereditary or environmental factors, or natural factors. A mix of the two is additionally possible.

For example, if one of your parents is an asthma or allergy victim themselves, then that boosts the odds that you might end up being a victim too. If both parents have an identical issue, then your odds of establishing asthma are considerably increased too.

Furthermore, there are lots of acknowledged environmental aspects or 'triggers' which could cause an asthma attack, with these triggers normally being broken down into 2 various categories.

The initial asthma trigger group would be those which trigger an allergic swelling of the air passages, with the triggers in this group called inflammatory triggers.

The second classification is that of non-allergic triggers that do not trigger the initial swelling. Nevertheless, they do have the capability to aggravate the victim, making them scratchy, which, consequently, could induce tension and anxiety that ultimately causes an asthma attack. These would be referred to as symptom triggers.

Inflammatory Triggers.

Animals: Remaining in near proximity to several kinds of animals, non-domesticated and domesticated, could induce an asthma attack. The following animals have been identified as having the capability to activate an asthma attack:

- Cats, the most typical cause

- Hamsters, mice and gerbils

- Rabbits

- Dogs

- And other 'furry' animals

It is typically thought that such an attack is set off by tiny dead skin particles from the animal being carried in the air. While this is partly correct, there are numerous other compounds which are created by animals, that could trigger an asthma attack, like saliva, physical secretions, and urine.

It is thought that up to half of kids who struggle with asthma are most frequently going to have an attack caused by close vicinity to animals. Even numerous kids who do not suffer serious asthma attacks are especially prone to environments where are a lot of animals.

Obviously, for numerous households, the cherished pet is a member of their family. However, if you choose to keep a pet, understanding that you are allergic or asthmatic to that pet, you are boosting your likelihood of suffering from asthma attacks with time. If you or a family members struggle with asthma, it is not advised to have furry pets in the house.

Dust mites: Dust mites are small bugs which live in identical spaces as people to feed upon the skin particles which people shed daily.

While you can discover dust mites nearly anywhere, even in the cleanest houses, they choose warm, wet environments where there is a lot of food offered. For this reason, the most typical locations to discover them would be soft, protected locations like bed linen, drapes, mats, carpets, cuddly toys, and soft, cloth-covered couches and chairs.

Even though it was normally thought up till just recently that lots of dust mites and house bugs (like the most typical, the bed bug) had actually been eliminated in Western nations like the U.S.A. and the UK, there has actually just recently been a considerable boost in the numbers of these pests residing in our houses. And while they are usually safe, they do shed body parts, which, along with their droppings, are understood to trigger the type of allergic reactions which could activate asthma attacks in specific individuals.

Molds: Molds are a kind of fungi discovered in nearly any dark, damp location. Molds don't, per se, trigger the type of allergic reactions that could cause an asthma attack, however, when they recreate, molds launch spores into the air as part of the procreation procedure, and these spores do trigger allergic reactions.

As recommended, molds are all over and are able to exist both inside and beyond the house. As a result, nearly anywhere or everywhere you go, you are subjected to mold spores, so you have to understand what actions to take to minimize your vulnerability to these spores.

Pollen: Pollens are commonly understood to be general irritants, triggering lots of medical conditions like hay fever. Pollen is a compound that triggers allergic reactions in lots of individuals all over the world. Regrettably, nevertheless, it is inconceivable to prevent it completely. Tree pollen is brought by dry, warm winds in the spring, grass and flower pollen are being transferred all over by the dry, hot wind in the summer season.

Cockroaches: Cockroach droppings have actually been revealed to activate asthma signs. If you reside in a location where cockroaches are an issue, the issue ought to be dealt with as soon as possible.

Viruses: Various kinds of viruses are understood to be behind setting off asthma attacks. They could additionally worsen the issue for anybody who is currently a victim of asthma. Viruses which trigger breathing problems, like the rhinovirus and other viruses which lead to the cold or influenza are most likely to be the ones which induce an asthma attack or make the condition worse.

Air Pollutants: Poor air quality renders it harder for anybody to breathe and can trigger a specific issue for anybody who is vulnerable to asthma. Industrial contaminants in the air we breathe are going to induce smog, whereas anything localized such as a greatly scented air freshener could be a severe issue for anybody who experiences asthma. Both of these substances could activate an allergic reaction, and they additionally have the capability to aggravate a pre-existing condition.

Asthma Triggers

Cigarette smoking: It is extensively acknowledged that cigarette smoke could activate asthma signs or set off an attack even in individuals who are not cigarette smokers themselves. Second-hand smoke is understood to induce asthma attacks.

Smoke is an irritant which assaults the internal lining of the breathing system, which is going to frequently set off an attack in anybody prone to asthma.

It is additionally commonly acknowledged that kids who are subjected to secondhand smoke are very likely to suffer much more asthma attacks, and those attacks are very likely to be much more serious.

If you or a member of the family are smoking cigarettes, while there are individuals in your home who are currently asthmatic or show indications of being asthmatic, it is suggested to stop cigarette smoking as rapidly as feasible.

Disregarding for a second all of the other advantages of giving up cigarette smoking, if you smoke somewhere where there is an asthmatic kid, you are substantially aggravating the kid's asthma condition needlessly.

Medications: A considerable percentage of individuals suffer allergic reactions to numerous extensively utilized medications like aspirin, and these medications can additionally induce an asthma attack.

Medicines like beta-blockers induce a contraction in the muscles which line the air passages. This tightness decreases airflow through the lungs and could aggravate or bring about an asthma attack.

Food allergies: Additionally, individuals who suffer allergic reactions to foods such as nuts or dry fruits are very likely to discover that their allergy can activate an asthma attack, with other typical allergies which induce issues consisting of gluten along with a response to seafood or eggs.

Antibiotic usage might promote asthma: Today, it is typical for antibiotics to be prescribed to deal with various medical conditions, and this applies just as much to really young kids as it does to grownups.

Nevertheless, research recommends that kids who go through an antibiotic course within the initial 6 months of their life are much more likely to establish allergies and asthma in later years than kids who have actually not been offered antibiotics. This is recommended on lots of well-respected sites such as WebMD.

This link is even more highlighted by the Department of Social Security in the UK along with the Health Department in Australia. Thus, there appears to be a probability that kids who take antibiotics in the initial 6 months of life are much more probable to establish asthma than those who do not.

Exercise: While exercise is usually something which is advantageous, it can induce issues for somebody who struggles with asthma, especially somebody whose asthma is not well managed.

Exercise induces issues due to the fact that, by definition, it boosts your requirement to take in additional air to sustain your efforts. Simultaneously, as a part of the workout, it is normal for your muscles to contract, so it is completely possible that your air passages are going to additionally contract at a time when you require them to broaden to be able to take more oxygen on board. Thus, exercise could be an issue for asthmatics.

Actually, you ought to see the issue the other way around. If exercise is resulting in problems, it most likely shows that your asthma is not adequately managed, suggesting it is time to do something about it. This is necessary since asthmatic or not, you do have to make routine exercise a part of your life to remain healthy.

Cold air, pollutants and fumes: As formerly discussed, incredibly cold air-- the sort which makes a non-asthma victim gasp for breath themselves-- is most likely to induce asthma-like signs in anybody who experiences the condition. Both very cold and hot air is outside the parameters or scope of the majority of people's typical environment, so both extremes can induce breathing troubles that may induce an asthma attack.

In the previous part, I pointed out that pollutants like smog could be both an inflammatory and a sign trigger. Harmful chemical fumes are sign triggers of asthma too.

While chemical fumes of this kind are not likely to be a huge issue for many people, there are particular locations like neighborhoods in close proximity to the chemical factory where fumes could be an asthma sign trigger. Furthermore, both pollutants and fumes could be an issue if they are present in your daily workplace. If feasible, you ought to make certain that you do not operate in a location where chemicals are to be utilized as a part of the regular daily regimen.

Pay attention to what you eat: Particular foods, specifically those which contain chemicals like monosodium glutamate, food additives (particularly tartrazine), and preservatives, are thought to have the capability to set off asthma attacks. Additionally, it is also normally suggested to stay away from foods that consist of mold or yeast like blue cheese, cakes, bread and beer as it appears that these compounds can additionally cause an asthma attack in specific people.

In addition, there is proof to support the suggestion that asthma is made worse by the rich diet plan more typical in industrialized Western nations as opposed to less industrialized nations elsewhere. Not just does the typical Western diet consist of much more treated and processed foods; however, Western diets additionally consist of less natural nutrients.

Proof for this originates from the reality that in lots of nations, individuals just started to establish asthma when they started to add western foods to diet plans to substitute those that they had actually generally consumed. For instance, up until the nation ended up being oil-rich and began importing Western foods, asthma was nearly unidentified in Kuwait. The identical phenomena additionally took place in New Guinea.

In Africa as well, a comparable pattern could be observed. As a matter of fact, in a letter which was released in the leading medical journal The Lancet, 2 scientists Neil and Keely reported on the 'Asthma Paradox' (p. 1099, 4/5/91) about kids in Zimbabwe by mentioning "... we discovered the occurrence of reversible air passages blockage to be 5.8% in richer metropolitan kids, 3.1% in poorer metropolitan kids, and 0.1% in rural kids." Reversible air passage restriction is one more medical term for asthma.

In Zimbabwe during the time, there was a huge distinction between the diet taken in by rural and metropolitan kids, once again implying that there is a link between a rich diet plan and the occurrence of asthma. Feelings and stress: Individuals who are susceptible to stress, anxiety or extreme feelings might as well discover that the beginning of any of these feelings or sensations might trigger an asthma attack.

There are numerous reasons why this might occur, like the truth that when we worry, we have a tendency to contract muscles. Contracting muscles in the chest might restrict respiratory tracts and place extra pressure on our lungs, leading to an asthma attack.

If you are the type of individual who's susceptible to anxiety attacks, emotional distress or stress, recognize that these could all make your asthma significantly worse and boost your danger of asthma attacks.

The List is Long

As you can see by now, the list of things which could cause asthma or cause an attack is a relatively long one.

This list is, in no way, thorough due to the fact that every single asthma victim is distinct. No doubt there are going to be certain individuals who struggle with asthma that read this who are exasperated or dissatisfied due to the fact that the #1 cause of their own asthma troubles is not included on this list, yet this just suggests the genuine nature of the issue.

While there are certain causes noted like smoking cigarettes that appear to trigger an asthmatic response in practically every victim, there are numerous other causes that might trigger an extremely major asthma attack in a single person and have no impact whatsoever on the next individual.

For instance, I have actually discussed a little handful of food allergies like nuts and foods which contain mold or yeast. There are potentially hundreds of other comparable allergies which could impact people and cause asthma attacks in sensitive people, while leaving other folks totally untouched.

This failure to figure out precisely what triggers asthma in different people can cause other troubles. For example, based upon the outcomes of some research, there are foods that are normally considered to be 'great' for you that might, however, hasten the advancement of asthma in kids.

One instance was highlighted in a heading from the New Scientist publication (19 July 2001): 'Margarine connected to dramatic asthma rise.'

The article included a report about the kids in 2 Australian towns who consume big quantities of polyunsaturated margarine and lower quantities of food fried in grease. These kids seemed two times as probable to establish asthma as kids who consumed less of these foods.

This might be taken to be verification that one of the essential fatty acids linoleic acid (Omega-6) might boost swelling, yet it opposes the notion that polyunsaturated margarine is a lot better for you than butter.

As a relatively severe instance, the BBC reported on their site numerous years ago that scientists in Belgium claimed that utilizing indoor swimming pools was among the reasons for the increase in asthma in kids, owing to the utilization of chemicals to clean the water.

The take-home message is that while lots of compounds, consisting of cleaning items and foods, have actually been suggested to be a causative factor in the advancement of asthma, there is no thing as an extensive list due to the fact that every person is distinct.

Can Asthma Be Cured?

The straightforward response to the question is no. There is no recognized remedy for asthma at the present time. The ideal method to deal with the condition is to manage it.

However, the bright side is that for a lot of asthma victims, managing their condition is a reasonably simple matter. With control, asthma patients could live a reasonably normal life with just a fairly tiny risk of asthma attacks happening.

For instance, I have actually already recommended that as soon as your asthma condition is under control, routine exercise is no tougher for an asthma victim as it would be for anybody else. Obviously, the following question is how to bring your asthma under control.

For the majority of people who experience asthma, the first individual to seek advice from is very likely to be their family doctor. Depending on your medical history, physical exam, and asthma symptoms and signs, your health care provider is going to suggest the ideal strategy to manage your asthma. Numerous asthma treatment strategies consist of medication as a means to manage asthma.

Similar to any other medical condition, there are additionally dangers associated with taking medications that are prescribed to address asthma.

Additionally, due to the fact that asthma is a chronic condition which can not be healed, any drugs that you so as to maintain your asthma under control are very likely to be drugs which you need to take for the remainder of your life. I will, for that reason, start our research on how you manage your asthma by looking at the conventional pharmaceutical drug-based approach.

Chapter 2: Drugs

Similar to any medical condition, if you believe that you or maybe your kid is demonstrating indications of asthma, you ought to look for a professional medical diagnosis right away. There is never any harm in looking for professional medical guidance, as it is constantly far better to understand precisely what the medical diagnosis is rather than supposing.

When you have actually consulted your doctor and have actually been diagnosed with asthma, it is very likely that they are going to propose an asthma action strategy which resolves the many problems associated with managing your condition.

It is additionally very probable that they are going to recommend a 2 phase approach for treating your condition utilizing pharmaceutical drugs. Generally, this includes 2 kinds of drugs, one that assists in stopping and managing asthma across the long run while the other is an emergency, fast relief option for when an asthma attack occurs.

Depending upon the usefulness of the long-lasting control program and the seriousness of your condition, it is very likely that the particular treatments and drugs which are going to be suggested are going to differ based upon the intensity of your condition. Additionally, when you go through particular life periods when things are changing fast, like menopause or pregnancy, your medications are going to have to be changed to mirror these life changes.

Nonetheless, the basic approach to managing asthma with pharmaceutical drugs constantly stays the same, which is utilizing a long-term drug to manage the condition and having a short-term emergency back-up to end an asthma attack when one takes place. We are going to look at every one of these in turn.

Chapter 3: Drugs for Long-Term Asthma Control

What They Are and How They Function

The most routinely prescribed medications for the long-lasting asthma control are corticosteroid drugs. Corticosteroids are anti-inflammatory medications. The main advantage of corticosteroids for asthma patients is they have the capability to decrease the odds of swelling in an asthma victim's breathing tract. Subsequently, they decrease the possibility of an inflamed air passage ending up being inflamed and causing an asthma attack.

Since the particular location of the body which is essential for an asthma victim is the respiratory tract, the majority of physicians would suggest taking inhaled corticosteroids for people struggling with asthma. This technique makes sure that the drugs are supplied to precisely the appropriate body part.

Numerous asthma victims who are initially introduced to the idea of breathing in corticosteroids daily for the remainder of their lives would be rather alarmed by the connection that they may create between anabolic steroids and these drugs. Nevertheless, the two drugs are entirely separate.

However, as you are going to find a bit later in this part of the book, corticosteroids resemble all medications because they do have prospective side effects, and a few of these side effects could be severe.

In many instances, specifically, if you struggle with serious asthma, your physician might advise taking corticosteroids by mouth as opposed to by inhalation. Undoubtedly, if you take the medications orally, more medication is going to enter into your bloodstream and be supplied to other parts of your body. Hence taking corticosteroids orally indicates that more medication is dispersed throughout your body, boosting the threat of undesirable side effects.

Other drugs which are often suggested as agents for long-term asthma management are as follows:

Long-acting beta2-adrenergic agonists: These are drugs which assist in opening your air passages that are usually taken in mix with inhaled corticosteroids as a means of avoiding and managing asthma signs in more serious cases. They must not be taken by themselves.

Leukotriene modifiers: These are drugs which are normally not considered to be as helpful as inhaled corticosteroids. Thus, they are usually recommended for individuals who suffer just moderate to mild asthma. Their function is to stop a lot of the physical responses which are a part of an asthma attack, like the restricting of the air passages and excess mucous.

Theophylline: This is one more drug which functions by unwinding the bronchial muscles to ensure that it frees up the respiratory tracts. It additionally has some acknowledged anti-inflammatory impacts too, which additionally improves its capability to clear the respiratory system, consequently making breathing less complicated.

Side Effects

As recommended above, many doctors choose to recommend inhaled corticosteroids, partly due to the fact that this makes sure that the drug goes to precisely the appropriate part of the body, and partly due to the fact that it additionally reduces the quantity of drug in the bloodstream and the resulting side effects.

Nevertheless, while corticosteroids are the most frequently assigned drug for asthma, they do have actually acknowledged side-effects. Corticosteroids could trigger cataracts, clouding the lens in your eye to ensure that your vision is going to weaken slowly. Keep in mind that this is a long-lasting drug that you are going to be on for the remainder of your life, so the odds of either cataracts or any of the other side-effects are very high to go up every year.

Another recognized side-effect of corticosteroids is osteoporosis, a steady deterioration of the bones throughout the years. Weaker bones undoubtedly render it even more probable that you are going to suffer dislocations and bone breaks in later life.

Moreover, it is additionally recommended here that corticosteroids could cause an even worse bone condition referred to as avascular necrosis. This is a condition where an absence of blood supply to bones in particular parts of the body can result in those bones, in fact, perishing.

Additionally, these identical sites recommend that long-lasting use of corticosteroids is probably going to result in irreparable thinning of the skin, rendering it even more probable that you are going to suffer an increasing number of injuries and skin lacerations as you age. Beneath this thinning skin, the blood capillaries are going to end up being a lot more exposed, making them much more susceptible to injuries and harm too.

Other side-effects which have actually been noted with particular corticosteroid brands are an overall rounding and rounding uo of the face ('moon face'), hypertension, headaches, weight gain, stomach ulcers, general muscle weakness, worsening of diabetes, childhood growth retardation, acne, and even psychiatric issues.

In 2005, the United States FDA released a notice that long-acting beta-2-adrenergic agonists had really raised the number of deadly asthma attacks in clinical trials. Specialists think that the reason for this was inappropriate utilization and prescribing of these medications. Long-acting beta-2-adrenergic agonists keep on being utilized today in mix with corticosteroids to protect against asthma attacks. Long-acting beta-2-adrenergic agonists must never ever be utilized throughout an intense attack. Short-acting beta-2-adrenergic agonists, like albuterol, are utilized to deal with acute asthma attacks and are gone over even more in the 'quick fix asthma drugs' part beneath.

Due to their fairly moderate nature, Leukotriene modifiers have not as yet shown any major negative side-effects.

Even though it used to be taken into consideration as one of the primary choices to deal with asthma, theophylline is no more consistently prescribed because of the danger of side severe side effects, tracking and interactions. Unfavorable impacts of theophylline consist of throwing up, stomach pain, headaches, diarrhea, irregular heart rhythms, seizures and others. Unlike other asthma drugs, theophylline calls for regular blood tracking. Theophylline additionally has lots of drug-food and drug-drug interactions which other medications that are successful at managing asthma do not.

Incorporating Natural Methods

Among the reasons why the long-lasting drugs that are most frequently prescribed for handling asthma have a lot of possibly undesirable side-effects is the cumulative nature of taking the drugs daily.

Subsequently, it shouldn't be a shocker that the possibly negative side effects are far higher from these longer-term drugs than they are from the quick fix emergency drugs which you are going to read about in the following chapter. Thus, all of the natural treatments which are going to be suggested later on are mostly targeted at substituting as many of the long-lasting drugs that you need to take to handle your asthma issue.

Additionally, in the worst-case scenario, asthma is an exceptionally harmful disease, one which could really kill you. It is, for that reason, most likely reckless to attempt to deal with each element of your asthma issue with totally natural treatments, since, in case of an abrupt, serious asthma attack, such treatments are not likely to be the most suitable.

Because of this, although I would advise that you attempt as many of the natural treatments for asthma as feasible, I would not always suggest that you discard the 'quick fix' emergency treatment which you are going to read about in the following part.

First of all, due to the fact that you utilize this 'quick fix' just in emergency situations, it is to be hoped that your use of it is exceptionally irregular, and for that reason, the adverse side-effects are highly probable to be marginal to non-existent. Second of all, you may have to utilize it to spare your life, and there could be no better reason than that.

Chapter 4: Quick Fix Asthma Drugs

The concept of the short-acting drug is that you have to have something which you are able to keep close by which you could utilize in the emergency situation.

Many people who struggle with asthma are, for that reason, very likely to bring a inhaler or nebulizer, which utilizes a short-acting beta2-adrenergic agonist drug which unwinds the muscles of the respiratory tracts and the chest really rapidly. In this way, the harshest results of an asthma attack could be countered within moments, making breathing simpler and unwinding the victim as a direct outcome.

As recommended in the previous chapter, long-acting beta2-adrenergic agonist drugs do have presumed side-effects, however, these side-effects are plainly going to be significantly less obvious in a short-acting drug which you just breathe in rarely in times of emergency situation.

Because of this, whilst I would suggest that you substitute long-acting beta2-adrenergic agonist drugs with natural treatments, I would not always claim that it is safe or suitable to do so with the short-term drugs which are utilized just when it comes to the emergency situation.

Chapter 5: Well-Managed Asthma

Peak Flow Meter

In case you're attempting to manage a long-term asthma issue, you want to have some method of understanding when you have that issue under control.

Due to this, you want to have a method of gauging your condition. The most reliable tool for self-assessing how effectively you manage your asthma is a peak flow meter, a tool which you could utilize at home to determine your optimum expiration rate of air or your peak expiratory flow rate.

Such a tool works for individuals who experience asthma due to the fact that by determining the quantity of air which you are breathing out, it could offer you a clear sign of how successfully you are breathing. As the performance of your expiration is straight related to how effectively your asthma is being managed, such a straightforward tool is all you actually require to determine your present control levels.

When utilizing such a peak flow meter, the initial thing which you want to do is developing a benchmark figure.

Over numerous days and, if at all feasible, during times when you are feeling unwinded and energetic, take a meter measurement. Take an average of these measurements throughout a number of days and utilize it as your regular or typical peak flow reading. You may, naturally, take the reading just one time; however, this risks entirely skewing the precision of your outcomes, so an average gathered over numerous days is much more beneficial.

With this benchmark developed, you ought to then take a routine measurement to compare your peak flow in particular conditions and at various times of the day with your baseline measurement. Utilize the next scale as an evaluation of your present condition of asthma control:

As pointed out previously, in case your asthma is appropriately managed, you ought to have the ability to do the majority of things which you would generally do, consisting of fairly strenuous exercise.

Nevertheless, whenever you do so, ensure that you take a meter reading fairly right after finishing your workout program since taking a measurement just when you are at rest and relaxed won't mean that much. Besides, if your asthma is under control, you undoubtedly wish to carry out typical daily activities, so you will not be doing anything except sitting around throughout the day.

In case your asthma is reasonably under control, you ought to have the ability to do 99.9% of what non-asthma patients may do, so testing in as many numerous conditions or circumstances is essential.

Spirometry

Spirometry is a more comprehensive method of measuring basically the identical things that utilizing a peak flow meter at home is going to measure, particularly the airflow in and out of your lungs and their performance.

Throughout this test that is going to normally be performed by your physician or a medical specialist, you will usually need to take a deep breath, clamp your mouth around the breathing tube on the device (referred to as a spirometer) prior to breathing out as much air as you are able to. Other tests which are in some cases carried out entail the patient breathing in and breathing out as strongly and rapidly as feasible, and in all instances, it is common to wear a nose-clip to make sure that you are just exhaling through your mouth.

Spirometry varies from utilizing a peak flow meter because it captures your whole forced breathing capability when measured versus time, while a peak flow meter is going to generally record the biggest breathing flow which you are able to sustain for 10 milliseconds.

A spirometer gauges your breathing capability in 2 ways, concentrating on:

- Forced expiratory volume (FEV1): This determines the air volume which you breathe out in the initial second of a forced exhalation.

- Forced vital capacity (FVC): Gauge the optimum volume of air which could be breathed out both by force and rapidly.

For an asthma victim, it is expected that the measurement applied to the breathing capability will be based upon the FEV1 reading. The figures beneath represent where you would stand in case you fell beneath 80% (of the standard for your weight, height, age, and gender) which would be taken into consideration as the lowest figure for an individual without any breathing troubles:

- FEV1 of between 61% and 80% of the typical figure indicates a mild breathing obstruction.

- FEV1 of between 41% and 60% of the typical figure indicates a moderate breathing blockage.

- FEV1 of less than 40% is a sign of a major or serious blockage which most likely requires attention as soon as possible.

Other Elements for Controlling Asthma

As it ought to be obvious by now, having your asthma under control is more related to the long-lasting nature of your issue than it is to the short-term asthma attacks which you may experience from time to time. Nevertheless, it ought to be obvious that the more regularly you suffer from these attacks, the more probable it is that your asthma is not as managed as you possibly believed it was.

As a basic guideline, if you do not suffer more than a couple of asthma attacks a week, you might presume that your asthma is under control. Taken together, excellent peak flow figures, fairly irregular asthma attacks and the capability to do nearly everything you wish to do would point to somebody who has their asthma well under control.

Nevertheless, understanding what you currently know about the possibly dreadful side effects of a few of the drugs which are typically utilized to manage asthma on a long-term basis, I would presume that you wouldn't always wish to attain this level of control utilizing these drugs. It is, for that reason, time to begin thinking about natural options.

Chapter 6: Changing Your Lifestyle

We have actually currently analyzed numerous elements which could activate asthma, varying from hereditary impacts about which you may do really little about to daily way of life elements like consuming unhealthy foods and smoking, which you could definitely do a good deal about.

Therefore, the very first aspect to think about is, what modifications can you make that are going to decrease the asthma risk in your life?

In order to this, you want to return to the earlier 'triggers' chapters to check out the list of aspects that may cause asthma or an asthma attack. In every instance, you want to ask yourself, is it likely that you could have an issue, and if so, could you deal with that issue?

There are certain changes which you could, without a doubt, incorporate practically instantly. For instance, if you consume dried fruit, nuts, and bread as part of your daily diet plan, you might attempt cutting them out to see if it makes any distinction. If it will make a distinction, it ought to be something which you would see inside a couple of days or weeks, either by utilizing your peak flow meter to register an enhancement in your quality of breathing or due to the fact that the regularity of asthma attacks drops off.

Do you read the labels on all the food which you consume? If not, then you are going to have little to no idea of whether you are consuming MSG, tartrazine, or any of the numerous various preservatives which are frequently utilized in daily foods. Begin reading the labels now and start to eliminate foods which have chemicals which might be a contributing element to your asthma.

If you have five furry animals running around your house, you ought to understand that they are worsening your asthma issue. Hence, you have a choice of residing with the issue or asking another person to care for your menagerie.

If you smoke, stop now. If another member of your household smokes, make them comprehend how ill it is making you in an attempt to get them to quit.

Even if you have the cleanest possible home, the odds are that you still have countless termites and bugs, and you might even have cockroaches. Call the regional pest control company immediately to get their help in eliminating these unwanted visitors.

Simultaneously, think about purchasing brand-new mattresses, bed linen, and pillows since eliminating the old things is among the fastest methods of cutting the population of unwanted 'visitors' by millions in one fell swoop. Have an eye on the pollen count in summertime and spring and attempt to stay clear of heading out any more than required when the figures are at their greatest.

In case you work in a job where you are exposed to chemical fumes or some other kind of contamination, is it reasonable to think about changing your work? If so, you need to do so, since it is apparent that your condition will never get better as long as you're doing work in a contaminated environment.

Are you an individual who experiences stress or anxiety attacks? If so, you may wish to think about taking up something such as yoga or meditation as a method of discovering how to manage your feelings. This, consequently, is going to minimize the probability that you are going to suffer repeating asthma attacks triggered by anxiety or stress.

In case you are consuming medication of some sort for another medical issue, are those medications worsening your asthma issue? If so, you ought to most likely speak with your medical attendant to see whether they are able to switch your medication to decrease the problems that the present medication is inducing you.

In case you have asthma, the way of life that you presently lead most likely plays a substantial role in making sure that you can not do away with your issue.

For this reason, making the required changes will be a considerable step in the appropriate direction, so you need to begin to make these modifications as rapidly as feasible.

Even in case each little change made just makes the smallest contribution to your efforts to decrease your vulnerability to asthma attacks, the mixed impact of all of these modifications taken together is going to be considerable.

Chapter 7: Natural Treatments

There are great deals of natural solutions which you could apply to minimize the intensity of your asthma issue. However, prior to heading any further, there is something to keep in mind.

Each asthma victim is distinct and, for that reason, it follows that what is effective for someone in curbing the intensity (and even doing away with) of their asthma may be entirely futile for somebody else. In other words, whilst anything that is going to be presented from this point on has actually been demonstrated to work for certain individuals, not everything is probable to work for you.

It is, for that reason, to a big degree, a matter of hit and miss. Attempt as many of the proposed ideas as feasible, go with every one of them for a couple of days or a week, and by the end of that time, re-assess your circumstance and condition.

Nevertheless, in case you follow a trial and error program, you ought to do so by testing only one compound or idea at a time.

It is just by testing that you can figure out precisely what it is that is working for you, whereas if you attempt mixing 3 or 4 recommendations together simultaneously, you are going to have far less of what is actually useful.

Multivitamins

Whilst we very likely all understand that if we ate a completely well-balanced diet plan, we would obtain all of the minerals, vitamins and other nutrients we require. However, for a lot of us, in the helter-skelter of daily life, it is genuinely challenging to consume such a perfect diet plan.

Subsequently, if you believe that your everyday diet plan is in any way out of balance or in some way lacking, you ought to think about taking a multivitamin daily.

If you do so, it is usually accepted that the vitamins that are most helpful in maintaining asthma at bay are B12 and B6, which is ideally mixed with folic acid for optimal asthma combating impact. However, you ought to stay clear of taking on board excessive magnesium and Vitamin C, in addition to excess quantities of fish-based items, which might include Omega-6, which was highlighted previously as a possible reason for asthma.

Honey

Honey is thought to be helpful in minimizing the occurrence of asthma attacks, especially when it is mixed with a natural anti-oxidant like turmeric extract or cinnamon powder.

If you choose to take honey by itself, then one teaspoonful daily suffices to offer alleviation from the worst impacts of asthma. If, however, you wish to optimize the usefulness of this specific natural treatment, then your first choice is to take in the teaspoon of honey with half a teaspoonful of cinnamon powder either initially in the early morning or final thing in the evening.

Additionally, you could warm a teaspoon of honey to ensure that it is actually warm prior to blending it with a quarter teaspoonful of turmeric powder, prior to taking in this potion two times daily.

Another thing which you may attempt is to hold a container of honey beneath the nose of somebody who is suffering from an asthma attack. In many instances, this could assist in reducing the victim's breathing by freeing up their respiratory tracts whilst additionally making it simpler for them to draw in a higher volume of air.

Nevertheless, in this last circumstance, I would still nonetheless ensure that you have their emergency nebulizer handy, simply in case this specific approach does not work in an emergency circumstance.

Garlic

Garlic could assist in reducing the majority of the signs of asthma and asthma attacks since the active components which provide garlic its natural pungent scent are additionally effective natural inflammatory compounds which assist in decreasing the propensity to suffer swelling that is an attribute of asthma.

So as to utilize garlic most successfully, boil 10 garlic cloves in half a pint of water between 5 and 10 minutes prior to consuming the liquid. Whilst boiling the garlic in this way is going to eliminate a great degree of the natural pungency of the veggie, it is going to still, nonetheless, stick around on your breath, so I would suggest that you consume this last thing prior to going to sleep if you do not wish to ruin your social life totally!

Additionally, attempt creating a ginger tea brew prior to including 2 cloves of garlic to your cup. This integrates 2 of the most effective natural anti-inflammatory compounds in one beverage, so by quaffing a cup of garlic-infused ginger tea initially in the early morning and the final thing in the evening, you ought to, once again, have the ability to lower the worst impacts of asthma.

Apple Cider Vinegar

Apple cider vinegar is one more option that is thought to have anti-inflammatory qualities, so you could either try a teaspoonful (it could be really sour or bitter) prior to each meal, or you could drop 2 tablespoonfuls into a glass of warm water prior to consuming one daily.

Get Rid of Dairy

Numerous asthma victims discover that eliminating or lowering dairy items from their diet plan entirely supplies a substantial increase to their efforts to lower the worst impacts of asthma. There are several reasons why this may be the case.

When it comes to cheese, you are taking a look at a dairy item which has actually been fermented, and for that reason, lots of cheese items are extremely abundant in yeast, which could be really bad for somebody who experiences asthma.

Milk-based items promote the production of mucous-- if you consume full-fat milk, you could nearly feel it taking place as you consume it-- and the final thing that any asthma victim requires is a food item that does this, due to the fact that they currently have ample issues with their own natural capabilities to generate more mucus than they require. If you take yogurt, even completely fat-free natural 'live' yogurt, you are receiving germs which may aggravate your body or trigger an unfavorable response.

Essentially, for numerous asthma victims, eliminating dairy items is something which aids them. It is, for that reason, something which you ought to think about if you have actually not currently done so.

Remove Wheat (Gluten) Based Items

Getting rid of wheat-based items from your diet plan ought to additionally supply your breathing capability with a considerable increase. Biscuits, cakes and commercially baked white flour bread ought to all be eliminated from your diet plan if at all feasible.

Drink Black Coffee

Whilst it may appear a little counterproductive to consume a caffeine-rich drink such as black coffee, it is, in reality, the caffeine in the beverage that renders it so valuable when it comes to fighting asthma. Caffeine is an effective anti-inflammatory agent, and for that reason, consuming black coffee could offer a considerable increase to your system's capability to hold up against the worst inflammatory attributes connected with asthma attacks.

Take Cold Showers

This one may sound a little 'bizarre' (i.e., insane), however, the truth is that taking core showers reinforces your immunity and encourages much better blood circulation, both of which are going to allow you to fight versus asthma even more successfully.

Simply taking one single cold shower daily can make an enormous distinction in your capability to withstand the worst devastations or impacts of asthma, so this is certainly something which is worth attempting due to the fact that proponents claim that the favorable outcomes are practically instantaneous!

Herbs

Along with ginger tea with its effective anti-inflammatory qualities, it is typically recommended that consuming natural teas like mint tea or chamomile could provide a substantial increase in your efforts to naturally beat asthma.

Many fans of organic teas claim that both mint and chamomile have the capability to unwind anybody who takes them regularly, along with having anti-allergenic qualities too.

If you're attempting to handle asthma, both these teas are well worth attempting since they could assist in minimizing the levels of tension and anxiety and stress in your daily life whilst additionally lessening the possibilities of the sort of allergies that are going to set off an asthma attack typically. It is additionally recommended that both of these herbs relieve your lymph nodes as well, which ought to once again assist in minimizing the odds of an asthma attack.

Other herbs which are thought to have anti-asthma qualities are lemon balm and sage, both of which are thought to have considerable recovery powers. Numerous other herbs are extensively thought to have effective antioxidant impacts, that are, once again, extremely handy in handling conditions where swelling is the norm, like asthma.

And whilst asthma itself is not a transmittable illness, we have actually currently seen that viruses could play an active part in triggering asthma attacks. Subsequently, the reality that much of the following herbs additionally have anti and antiviral-bacterial properties makes them much more important to an asthma victim:

Rosemary: Rosemary activates your immunity, improves blood circulation, and enhances your food digestion. It additionally consists of precisely the type of anti-inflammatory substances that you require to combat asthma. Add to this the reality that it includes polyphenols, which are extensively acknowledged to be among the most powerful natural antimicrobial and antiviral substances, and you could see that rosemary is a really effective herb that could play an essential part in your battle versus asthma.

Oregano: It is thought that the antioxidant capabilities of the natural chemicals in oregano are up to 20 times more effective than those of any other herb. It additionally has powerful microbial qualities along with being an abundant source of much of the vitamins which you require in a well-balanced diet plan. Include this to the reality that it consists of omega-3 fats, and you have another herb which you ought to incorporate in your everyday diet plan (it's awesome on pasta and pizzas particularly).

Dill: Dill is yet another herb with recognized antioxidant qualities which additionally supplies a considerable calcium source, consequently protecting from bone loss. It is additionally an abundant source of trace elements like magnesium, manganese, and iron, all of which you require as part of a healthy diet plan which you need to consume in your natural fight versus asthma.

Tarragon: Tarragon belongs to the daisy and dandelion family, a herb which is once again exceptionally abundant in anti-oxidants in addition to anti-inflammatory and anti-bacterial agents. Moreover, it assists with reinforcing your immunity and shielding your liver simultaneously.

Motherwort: Motherwort is a herb which is extremely reliable for opening the air passages naturally, along with having the capability to unwind anybody who takes it so that anxiety and stress, which could worsen asthma, are both reduced.

All of the herbs noted above could assist in your battle versus asthma. Nevertheless, herbs on their own are not a magic bullet which is going to remove your issue overnight.

However, by boosting the number of herbs you take as part of your daily diet plan whilst following the other dietary standards in this book, you are going to be doing a lot to increase your body's capability to fight asthma.

A Natural Asthma Eating Plan

Along with much of the foods pointed out earlier and the herbs discussed in the last part, among the most reliable methods of combating asthma is to ensure that your body is as healthy and strong as feasible. So as to do this, you want to consume a diet plan for strength and health.

Therefore, you ought to base your diet plan on the following standards:

- Consume lots of fresh vegetables and fruits, preferably raw, yet steamed if they need to be cooked;

- Take it easy with the red meats, and eliminate dairy items as formerly discussed;

- Have an eye on your fat intake, since a low-fat diet plan is, without a doubt, more preferable than the one high in fats;

- Include garlic, ginger and onion, however, withstand the urge to cook the heck out of them, due to the fact that when you do, you additionally cook out the good stuff;

- Wheatgrass juice is fantastic for eliminating contaminants and lowering the quantity of mucus in the body;

- Attempt to fast one day a week where you consume just raw vegetables and fruits. If you can do so, it is going to considerably lower both the contaminants and mucous in your body, therefore decreasing the odds of asthma attacks.

Particular foods which you ought to feature in your diet plan as often as possible consist of grapes, bananas, oranges, spinach and bitter gourds along with all the things formerly pointed out.

All of these foods items offer a terrific source of nutrients and vitamins with numerous qualities which would assist an asthmatic manage their condition by maintaining the lungs lubricated, boosting amino acids that are anti-allergic for asthmatics, and so forth.

Chapter 8: Less Known Natural Options

Halotherapy or Speleotherapy

Have you ever delighted in that terrific sensation when you're standing beside the ocean, clearing your nostrils with the salt-laden air of the ocean?

In case you have, then you most likely currently value that breathing in salt enriched air is an extremely reliable method of enhancing your breathing in precisely the way you would wish to do in case your breathing is restrained by asthma.

You may, for that reason, wish to think about getting a salt inhaler, a tool with which you could breathe in air which passes over sea or mountain crystal salt.

Certainly, the tool works on precisely the identical principle as does the ancient 'folk' remedy of clearing the worst impacts of influenza or cold by breathing in the fumes from hot saltwater, which is a variation of a treatment which has actually been utilized since ancient times. Undoubtedly, salt treatment was proposed by Hippocrates, who is usually taken into consideration as the father of contemporary medicine over 2000 years back, so it could hardly be claimed to be a new idea.

Nonetheless, there does appear to be a lot of proof that utilizing salt treatment by doing this might be something which might prove to be a huge aid in your efforts to decrease the worst impacts of asthma in an absolutely non-invasive and natural manner.

Marine Phytoplankton

In recent times, certain researchers have actually demonstrated that marine phytoplankton might suffice by itself to combat the worst impacts of asthma.

Due to the fact that phytoplankton is commonly taken into consideration as the source of all life in the world-- according to NASA, it generates 90% of the oxygen we inhale-- and due to the fact that phytoplankton have actually been populating the oceans for more than 300 million years, it's probably not unexpected that the environment wherein phytoplankton live is a strikingly close match to the structure of human cells.

Subsequently, researchers are now working on the theory that phytoplankton might provide a solution to much of the most intractable medical issues humanity has actually ever needed to deal with, while maybe being able to supply us with a natural remedy for a wide variety of conditions such as asthma.

The recommendation is that a teaspoon of phytoplankton material daily may be adequate to treat existing illnesses and fend off future medical disasters.

The only issue is, phytoplankton is reasonably challenging to draw out from its surrounding environment-- maybe not too unexpected when you realize that plankton are nearly undetectable even under the most strong microscopic lense-- so if you can discover phytoplankton to purchase, it is most probably going to be excessively pricey. Nonetheless, with the extremely genuine possibility that we may be able to 'farm' phytoplankton in the fairly near future, there is a real possibility that an absolutely natural 'remedy' for asthma is not all that far off.

Embracing a Homeopathic Approach to Dealing With Asthma

When any kid or grownup suffers from an asthma attack, we have actually currently established that they are going to generally be treated with a nebulizer, and that provides a quick 'blast' of inhaled drugs. Any attack like that begins when something has actually activated it, so the homeopathic approach claims that this trigger is not just part of the disease, yet additionally part of the remedy.

The homeopathic technique intends to tap into the body's own capability to recover itself by making the trigger part of the cure, on the basis that stopping the signs is inadequate. Asthma homeopathy takes the view that in order to deal with asthma properly, you need to deal with the patient's entire body simultaneously, as you can not separate one single cause from the entirety.

Simultaneously, even homeopathic specialists who specialize in dealing with asthma comprehend that there is no single treatment which works extremely well for everybody since each person's asthma case is distinct.

The homeopathic method of dealing with any specific medical condition is to deal with that condition as if it is a sign of something which is wrong with the entire organism, instead of being the issue in itself. And there appears little doubt that for some people, embracing the homeopathic approach towards asthma is going to work. There are, for instance, reports that claim that utilizing homeopathy to handle asthma has actually led to certain people establishing boosted immunity that have allowed them to fight versus the illness totally naturally with no additional external support.

Regrettably, there is a relative scarcity of top quality information regarding homeopathic asthma treatment on the web, so if this is a manner of handling your issue that you want to consider, attempt looking for a regional homeopath with whom you are able to talk about your issue and any options that they may be able to provide.

Conclusion

Asthma is a horrible issue which is suffered by numerous individuals all across the world, even though there does appear to be a greater frequency of asthmatics in industrialized nations where the diet plan is richer than there are in less industrialized nations. However, for asthma victims all across the world, it is an issue which is at best frightening and incapacitating, whilst at worst, it could be deadly.

As recommended, if you think that you have an asthma issue, you want to go to an accordingly certified doctor to look for diagnostic verification. Afterward, you have some choices, however, in all sincerity, I would claim that there truly are no choices.

We have currently established that a number of the drugs which are recommended for long-lasting control of asthma could have certain extremely undesirable side effects, whereas there are no evil side-effects when it comes to natural options.

Considering that each asthma victim responds to treatments in various ways and the truth that a lot of these natural approaches of dealing with asthma have actually been verified to work, it makes sense to attempt to handle your asthma condition naturally prior to looking to pharmaceutical drugs.

What you do for short-term treatment is going to hinge on how severe your asthma attacks are, since if they are severe enough, you might still have to utilize a nebulizer. However, over the long run, embracing a natural approach to handling your asthma issue has actually got to be the practical method of dealing with things.

I hope that you enjoyed reading through this book and that you have found it useful. If you want to share your thoughts on this book, you can do so by leaving a review on the Amazon page. Have a great rest of the day.

Printed in Great Britain
by Amazon